How to Lose Weight While Playing with Your Kids

Tyler Buckhouse Copyright © 2015

Disclaimer

How to Lose Weight While Playing with Your Children

If you're a parent, you know how hard it is to find time to eat healthy and to exercise, especially if your children are younger. Children take up the majority of your time and attention which makes it difficult to get in a workout, especially one that is effective and burns calories in order to shed those unwanted pounds.

Having kids may also mean fast food and junk food in the house, as these are often favorites of most children. Of course, the grownups can't help but to share in the indulgences. Sugary foods and sodas, deep fried foods, and snacks that are just empty calories can cause parents to pack on the pounds quickly and easily.

For any parent who are struggling with their weight and wonder if the situation is hopeless or at least unchangeable until their children leave home, there is good news. You can actually lose weight despite the time and attention that your children need. You can even use time with them as a way to help you lose weight.

The keys to successfully losing weight with your children include knowing how and why you gain weight in the first place, and then using that information to your advantage when you are with your children. Many people have a basic understanding of how food and physical activity affect your weight and are often times misguided about body weight.

To better understand how you can lose weight when with your kids, you first need to consider some basic information about body weight, metabolism, nutrition, and activity. This will ensure that you apply all of the information effectively, and understand why certain changes may need to be made to your routine and overall eating habits.

HOW YOU GAIN AND LOSE WEIGHT

Your body weight is a result of the calories that you consume versus the calories you burn off through physical activity. There are other factors involved, but those other factors are still related to your calorie consumption versus calories burned.

UNDERSTANDING CALORIES

Because your body weight is a balance of calories consumed versus burned, it's good to know what calories are in the first place. A calorie is not a physical element of food like vitamins or trace minerals, but it is a way of measuring potential energy in food. The more calories in food, the more potential energy it will provide to you.

The body stores any unused potential energy as body fat, to be used later when you need to be physically active but don't have an energy source. The body also stores fat as a way to protect itself when food supplies run low. The more calories you ingest but don't burn off through activity, the more body fat you'll store.

To cut down on the body fat you store, you need to create a balance of the calories you consume versus the ones you burn off. You can consume fewer calories, be more physically active, or both. To lose one pound of body fat, you need to actually burn some 3500 calories more than you ingest.

UNDERSTANDING METABOLISM

Many people use the word metabolism and they know that it plays a role in weight loss. However, they don't really understand what it actually is. It's vital to know about metabolism if you want to lose weight and keep it off for good.

What is a metabolism?

Your metabolism is the average rate at which you burn calories throughout the day. When you're physically active you're burning more of that potential energy measured as calories, and when you're at rest your body is still using energy to keep its major systems functioning but not as much. Your metabolism is the average number between these two extremes.

When you burn more calories per day than the average person, it is considered a high or fast metabolism. When your metabolism is less than average, it is a slow or low metabolism. Increasing or speeding up your metabolism will allow you to burn more calories every day so that you store less body fat and use up the fat reserves you have.

Improving your metabolism.

There are a few different ways of improving your metabolism. One is to be more physically active. This helps you to burn more calories as you're being active but even while you're at rest. The reason for this is that your body still works hard after you've been physically active so you're still burning calories. The muscles you use during activity need to be restored and repaired from their exertion. The body is pumping blood through your system even after you stop being active, since it is a healing agent. This blood carries healing oxygen, and your lungs keep working after you've been active to bring more oxygen into your body.

You may notice that this is true. After a good jog or bike ride, you can still feel your heart beating and your lungs pumping more actively than usual. Once you stop jogging or get off your bike, your heart rate and breathing don't immediately drop to normal levels! You're burning more calories even after a good workout, so being physically active is a good way to improve your metabolism.

Another way to improve your metabolism is to build and improve muscle tone. The body needs to work constantly to support muscles as they need to be fed and repaired. The body does not need to work as hard to support fat. Bodybuilders will have a naturally higher metabolism than anyone else because their body is working even when they're at rest to support those muscles. When you exercise, you need to do aerobic activity to burn calories but resistance training will also help you to lose weight and stay slim.

UNDERSTANDING TYPES OF FOOD AND WEIGHT GAIN

Along with a lack of information and misconceptions about calories and metabolism, many people also have incorrect ideas about food and how it affects your body weight. Counting calories alone is not the solution to losing weight and keeping it off. You need to understand how food affects your body so you can make healthier choices that will help you with your weight loss goals. The right food choices can fill you up and energize you while providing you with fewer calories. Unhealthy food choices can cause you to pack on the pounds without giving you the nutrition and energy that you need.

Sugar and hunger.

You should try to avoid sugar as much as possible when trying to lose weight because it's just empty calories. Sugar has no nutritional value and does nothing in your system. It only causes you to pack on the pounds. However, the calorie content of sugar is not its only concern when it comes to weight loss.

When you eat sugar, it gets ingested in the bloodstream. When blood sugar levels go up, the body creates hunger pains. This is because it needs insulin to even out those sugar levels, and the pancreas releases insulin when you eat. This reaction is one reason why a person often feels hungry after eating sugary foods. You are not really hungry for food. Your body is trying to force you to eat so that it can have the needed insulin.

Understanding carbohydrates.

There are two types of carbohydrates found in foods; simple and complex. Complex carbohydrates are difficult to break down and give you energy. They are found in unprocessed grains and foods that are high in fiber content.

Simple carbohydrates have been processed so that most of the grains are removed. This includes anything made with white flour or white rice. They also include starchy vegetables such as potatoes.

One reason that carbohydrates have gotten such a bad reputation with dieters in the past few years is that they break down as sugar in the body. They are not only very calorie-dense but they cause the blood sugar levels to spike. This causes a person to feel hungry after eating simple carbohydrates.

Protein and hunger.

When trying to lose weight, eating more protein is always recommended. This is because protein has a chemical that sends a signal to the brain, telling it that the stomach is full. Other foods do not have this chemical. You can easily overeat simple carbohydrates and sugar without ever feeling full. However, it's very difficult to overeat when you have protein. Eating more protein can help to control your hunger while you try to cut calories.

The importance of fiber.

Most people know that fiber makes you regular in the bathroom. It has many other benefits and is a very important part of the diet of those wanting to lose weight. Fiber expands and absorbs water as it's digested, so it helps you to feel full. You can fight off hunger pains when you eat fiber. You may find that you eat less overall.

Fiber also binds to other foods and helps them to break down so they get more readily absorbed into the system. You'll be ingesting more healthy vitamins and trace minerals from your foods when you eat enough fiber. This supports physical activity better by providing you with more energy. You may also find that you will suffer from fewer illnesses.

Calorie-dense foods.

One reason that many people feel hungry when they're trying to lose weight is that they eat calorie-dense foods. As a result, they don't each much but are still take in many calories. Calorie-dense foods have a high amount of calories for a small amount of food. Switching to foods that are less calorie dense will allow you to eat more and lose weight.

To illustrate what is meant by calorie-dense foods, consider a boneless skinless chicken breast. Half of a breast is 86 grams or 3 ounces. It contains 141 calories and no carbohydrates. However, a 3 ounce commercially prepared muffin has over 300 calories and nearly 70 grams of carbohydrates. You can see how the same amount of food has over twice the calories!

If you choose foods that are not as calorie-dense, you can either eat less food or you can eat the same amount of food, feel full and still be getting fewer calories.

PHYSICAL ACTIVITY AND WEIGHT LOSS

Now that you have a better understanding of how food choices affect your overall body weight, you need to think about your physical activity levels and the types of activities in which you engage so that you can lose weight. Similar to food, not all physical activities and exercise methods are created equal. They won't all help you to lose weight and keep it off. While all forms of activity will burn calories, some burn such a small amount of calories that they will have little impact on your overall body weight.

The benefits of interval training.

Interval training refers to physical activity that changes every few minutes, either changing the part of the body being exercised or the intensity levels. An example of interval training might be to walk for a few minutes to warm up, sprint as fast as you can, jog lightly, sprint again, walk again, and repeat this cycle. Each speed lasts for only a few minutes.

As another example of interval training would be to do some jumping jacks to warm up and bench press a few sets, do more jumping jacks, an arm pull-down exercise, a quick set of leg presses, and then repeat this cycle.

Each of these activities has a benefit because it keeps the body guessing. When you walk, sprint and walk again, your heart and lungs are being challenged to their max. When you use interval training to train different muscles one right after another, none of them become accustomed to what you're doing and in turn, exert less effort. When you change up your routine, your muscles are being challenged to their max so they're working as hard as they can. As a result, you're burning the maximum amount of calories.

The benefits of resistance training.

Resistance training refers to workouts that build and tone muscles rather than just burn calories. Lifting weights, using weight machines and exercise bands, and intense Pilate routines all build and firm muscles.

The body works harder to support muscle than it does fat. Therefore, if you have good muscle tone, you will be burning more calories every minute of the day, even when at rest. There's no need to worry about getting too big and muscular, which is a common concern for women. Bodybuilders and those you see in fitness competitions usually work out for several hours every day. They lift enormous amounts of weight that would be impossible for average people to lift. Steroid use is also common among professional bodybuilders. Therefore, you should focus on how you can incorporate resistance training into your routine.

High impact versus low impact aerobic routines.

High impact routines refer to exercises that pick your feet up off the ground; you then impact the ground as you step back down. As a result, your entire body feels this impact or shock. Low impact or no impact routines refer to those where you don't pick up your feet. This may include riding a bike or using an elliptical machine. It could also involve a routine like Pilates where you step up simply to change positions and don't actually impact the ground.

The benefit of high impact aerobic routines is that they typically burn more calories since you need to exert more effort. Every time you lift your feet high enough to create this type of impact, you are actually fighting the force of gravity. The drawback is that your entire body absorbs this impact and these routines can cause damage to your knees, back, and other joints. Low impact routines can still burn calories and build muscle tone if you exert enough effort during those routines and use enough resistance. However, they need to be challenging in order to have the same benefit.

LOSING WEIGHT WITH YOUR KIDS

You now have a basic understanding of how the body gains and loses weight and what it takes to shed unwanted pounds and keep them off. This information can be used and applied to spending time with your kids. There is general information about how to stay active when you're with your kids, and specific information about creating opportunities to stay active and eat healthy when you are with your children.

BEING ACTIVE WHEN WITH YOUR KIDS

Being active when you're with your kids boils down to simply choosing to be active rather than passive with them.

Choosing to be active.

Consider some simple tips when it comes to getting up and being active with your kids rather than sitting back and watching them play:

- When you're at the playground, do you actually play with the children or sit on a bench while they play? To stay active, get up and push your children on the swings, help them down the slide, or run with them around a play set.

- Help them clean their room and the house rather than just sending them to do certain chores. You can make a game out of it by seeing who can do their list of chores faster. You'll be more active and will also set an example for them about getting up off the couch.

- Choose active rather than passive video games. Many game consoles use paddles to simulate real games such as bowling or tennis, or you might find dancing games you can play with your kids rather than standard shooting or action games.

- Choose active toys for your children so that you can play together. Even smaller children can use a plastic basketball hoop you set up in the living room, or you might choose a plastic bowling ball and pin set. While building blocks and puzzles are good choices, be sure you balance these with games that you can play with your children while being active.

- If you take your child to an arcade, encourage him or her to play some of the more active games and get up and play with them. Even if you stand up while they play other video games, this will be more active than sitting back and watching them play on their own.

- Walk or ride your bikes to the corner store when you need bread or milk, rather than driving there. Walk with your child to a friend's house rather than driving him or her there, if it's just a few blocks away.

Creating active opportunities.

Being active with your kids doesn't always happen by chance. As a parent you may need to create opportunities to be active with them. If you choose fun activities, your children may be more receptive to the idea of getting off the couch and turning off the television. Consider some suggestions for how to do this:

- Get good bikes for yourself and the kids. If you cannot afford new bikes, check out resale shops, online classified ads, and other places where you can get used bikes. A bike should last for years. Even a used bike should be a good investment for you and your children. Remember that you don't need to take your bikes to a special path or park to enjoy them. You can get into the habit of riding around your neighborhood after dinner. This can help everyone in the family to burn calories.

- If you can, invest in a basketball hoop for your driveway or to install over your garage door. Play a game with your kids for an hour every night.

- A badminton set is very affordable and doesn't take up much space outdoors. It is a game that just about everyone in the family can play.

- Play follow-the-leader indoors or outdoors, and take turns being the leader. Get creative with where you go in the house to give yourself a thorough workout. You can crawl under the dining room table or get out a stepstool and use it to walk over. You can get creative with movements to add to this game for even more of a workout. You can do somersaults in the living room or try doing cartwheels or handstands outside.

- Try a variation of follow-the-leader by marching around the home or your yard. Marching kicks your feet up higher than simple walking and may help you to burn more calories.

- Remember that games don't need to be fancy and equipment doesn't need to be expensive for kids to enjoy them and to keep everyone active. Toss a ball back and forth or kick one back and forth across your yard. You can also play with a Frisbee outside or at the park. Use a hula hoop and have a contest to see who can hula the longest. Put on some music and have a "Dance Off," with everyone showing off their fanciest moves.

Exercising with your kids.

Kids should never be made to feel fat or ugly or otherwise unattractive. However, exercise routines can be fun if they're presented as being enjoyable or as a game. Pilate moves are fun for kids and can build strong muscles. You can also try normal exercise moves with your kids if you make them fun. Consider some simple Pilates moves and other exercises you might try with your kids and how to make them enjoyable for both of you.

- The swim is a great choice for Pilates and builds a strong core. To perform this movement, lie on your stomach with your arms outstretched, legs behind you and feet slightly apart. Move your arms and legs up and down as if you're slapping water. Make a game of it by telling your kids you're trying to get across a lake or are pretending that you have a pool.

- Rolling like a ball is also fun for kids. To perform this movement, sit up and pull your knees to your chest, hugging your arms around your legs. Gently pick your feet up off the floor. Your stomach muscles will contract to support your weight and you can gently roll from side to side or back and forth. This is a great movement for kids on its own.

- Figure eights are also fun for kids. Lie on your back with your legs straight in the air, feet together. Gently move your legs at the hips to make figure eights in the air, keeping your legs in a tight circle so they don't go past your hips. This will also build strong abdominal muscles, and kids will love the movements as well. Make it a game by asking them to write words in the air and take turns guessing what you're writing.

- A good variation of this game is to use just one leg. Keep one leg on the ground and rotate the other leg slowly in the air. This can be easier for those who don't have the strength to support both legs.

- Sit-ups can be fun with your kids. Lie down on the floor, next to each other with your feet tucked under the couch. Hold a ball in your hands, and as you both sit up, hand the ball to your child. As he or she reclines and then sits up, they hand the ball back to you. Take turns, and then see how quickly you can do this without dropping the ball or missing a handoff.

- Rolling forward can also create strong back and gluteus muscles and they're fun for kids as well. Lie on your stomach with your head and back curved up, arms straight out in front of you. Roll forward as you lift your legs and continue to roll back and forth, alternating between your legs and with your upper torso balancing you.

Remember that very often, burning calories and being active with your kids is simply a matter of being creative and taking the initiative. Look for ways to get up and move around with them, and for ways to make it fun to be active with them.

EATING HEALTHY WITH YOUR KIDS

Making healthy eating choices with your kids can be a challenge since kids usually love sugar, fat, and empty calories of all sorts. Families also may struggle to find the time to prepare healthy foods and may rely on fast foods, frozen foods, and foods that are quick and easy. Unfortunately, this often means pasta choices like macaroni and cheese and spaghetti, or other choices that are going to pack on the pounds.

Eating healthy with your kids to lose weight and keep it off is much like being active; it simply takes preparation and determination. You don't always need to spend hours each day to prepare healthy food choices and you can still enjoy the occasional treat while losing weight. Consider some tips on how to do this.

Learning to use tools and simple cooking techniques.

Very often simple cooking techniques and the right tools can make healthier eating options easy for you. Consider a few examples of how this can work in your home, even if you're busy with your kids:

- Investigate marinades for lean protein choices like chicken breasts and lean pork chops. Use an indoor grill so you can cook these simply and quickly and don't need to rely on frying to add flavor. You can put the chicken or pork in a bowl with the marinade before you go to bed, and the next day it's fully saturated and ready for the grill when you walk through the door after work.

- A slow cooker or crock-pot can cook a healthy meal without much effort. You can put a chicken in the slow cooker in the morning along with some seasoning, and at night have a hot meal ready for dinner without using extra oils for flavor and without taking extra time for cooking.

- A crock pot is also good for making homemade soups and chili, which in turn allows you to control the ingredients. Make a homemade vegetable soup or vegetarian chili on the weekend and then freeze individual portions so you have a quick meal option during the week. When you make homemade options, you can use spices to add flavor and don't need to rely on added fat and sugar that is common with canned soup and chili.

- A rotisserie can make a great meal without using oils for frying. Add seasoning to your chicken or pork loin and it will baste in its own juices, making it a healthier choice than deep frying.

Opt for healthier alternatives.

Sometimes just making a few simple changes can allow you to eat healthy without missing out on your favorite flavors and snacks. Consider a few tips:

- If your kids love crispy snacks like potato chips and pretzels, try a healthy alternative by slicing a potato very thin, adding seasoning, and cooking it at high temperatures for several minutes. Baked potato chips have much less fat and fewer calories than standard chips.

- Make baked apples for dessert with just a sprinkle of cinnamon rather than cake or ice cream or any other high-calorie treat.

- Choose turkey burgers or vegetarian burger rather than regular hamburger. These both have fewer calories and less fat overall.

- Instead of chips and dip for a snack, opt for vegetables with hummus or ranch salad dressing as a dip. These both have fewer calories and less fat, and the vegetables are a much healthier alternative to potato chips.

- Remember to always use fruit as a snack rather than anything sugary when you need to satisfy your sweet tooth. Apples and bananas are high in sugar so opt for berries, grapes, and melons instead. These are better for cutting calories and helping you to lose weight.

- Look for healthy cereals rather than sugary choices that are just empty calories. Choose those that are high in fiber and low in calories. Bran cereals are good, or you might opt for oatmeal with a bit of fresh fruit and cinnamon rather than cold cereal.

- Soy milk and almond milk have less fat and fewer calories than dairy milk. Unsweetened almond milk has 30 calories per cup, versus 120 calories for skim dairy milk! Switch to either soy or almond milk for everyday use to easily cut hundreds of calories every week, and chances are your kids won't notice the difference.

Adding healthier choices to your diet.

To be healthy and to lose weight, you must not only cut out unhealthy options but also fill up on healthier choices for your everyday eating. This is how you can do this with your kids:

- Oatmeal can add fiber to your diet and help you feel full. Get into the habit of making instant oatmeal for breakfast every morning. You can heat up a bowl of instant oatmeal in the microwave in about two minutes with a small spoon of honey and some cinnamon. .

- Rather than peanut butter and jelly sandwiches, pack sandwiches for your child's lunch with lean lunchmeat options. Turkey and lean cuts of ham have more protein and no sugar, making them better options than peanut butter and jelly. The protein in the lunchmeat can help to fill them up through the afternoon.

- Add lots of lettuce, tomato, sprouts, cucumbers, and other vegetables to sandwiches. This not only helps to make you and your children feel full but it also means getting those healthy vitamins and trace minerals in your diet that these foods provide.

- Steam vegetables for side dishes for dinner rather than potatoes and other less healthy options. This will also help you to feel full and provide you with healthy vitamins and minerals.

- Have vegetarian dishes as often as possible, to avoid the fatty choices of red meat and pasta for dinner. Learn to cook stuffed peppers or use portabella mushroom as a main course. You can also prepare a plate of steamed vegetables with spice blends for a nutritious lunch on the weekends.

PUTTING IT ALL TOGETHER

If you're serious about losing weight with your kids, you will want to put all this advice together for the most benefit. It's not enough to just be active with your kids while you still fill up on sugary foods, or to cut down on sugary foods while still being inactive.

A good way to incorporate all these points is to note which ones you can use immediately and then continue to add in various points over the weeks. This week you might switch to almond milk and have lean protein choices for lunch while starting a simple Pilate routine with your kids. Next week, keep up these changes and then get a crock pot and a basketball hoop you can use regularly. The following week, learn how to cook vegetarian dishes. Each week you can make one small change and use one tip for increasing activity and eating healthier with your kids. You'll soon see the weight melting off and will notice that you can keep it off as well!

Remember that you can get your kids involved directly. Tell them that you're challenging yourself to make these changes and ask for their help to keep you on the straight and narrow. Ask them what changes they want to make when it comes to being active and exercising, and for their suggestions on games you can play to stay active. You may be surprised at how easily your kids can be convinced to help you with your weight loss goals and help you to keep the weight off!